Nostalgia

Famous Faces

SERIES EDITOR: Una P Holden
RESEARCHERS: Francesca Eason and Jo McCulloch

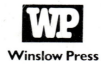

WP

Winslow Press

First published in 1985 by Winslow Press
23 Horn Street, Winslow, Buckingham MK18 3AP

Copyright © Winslow Press 1985

Designed & Printed by Redesign 01-533 2631

ISBN 0 86388 029 0

Credits

*The Editor is indebted to the BBC Hulton Picture Library
for the use of all photographs except the following:
Louis Armstrong, W.C. Fields, Charles de Gaulle,
Marilyn Monroe, Ronald Reagan and Edward G.
Robinson, all from The Bettmann Archive Inc.,
136 East 57th Street, New York, NY 10022 Plaza 8-0362.*

Contents

Nostalgia

This series of photo packs has been produced as an aid for group leaders working with elderly people. The purpose of the photographs is threefold:

(i)   to evoke memories of the past

(ii) to encourage people to recall and reflect on their own experiences in the past through pictures of objects, events and personalities

(iii) to provide a stimulus for group discussions and informal conversation between elderly people

Reminiscence in itself is believed to be therapeutic in that it arouses people's interest and attention and calls upon their store of knowledge and experience, and this in turn facilitates communication. The *Nostalgia* series of photographs provides a means for group leaders to focus attention on particular topics and will thus encourage elderly people to reminisce over specific times and events. The pictures can be used to develop discussion in a group or may usefully be given to two people to look through and chat about themselves.

The notes in this booklet give historical information relating to the subject of each photograph. The group leader will find it useful to have a few facts to refer to when developing the particular discussion theme.

The group leader may like to supplement the photographs with other material from the era such as objects, songs, records, equipment, books and any other available pictures relating to the topic on the card. In addition, members of the group should be encouraged to bring items from home to show to the rest, thus providing a focus to share memories of times past with each other.

It would also be useful if the leader could provide a few current newspapers, magazine cuttings and modern objects when possible to encourage comparison between past and present.

Famous Faces

This pack of photographs shows a selection of well-known people who achieved fame between the years 1920 and 1960. The selection has been made to provoke pleasant memories and provide as many talking points as possible. To encourage conversation about these well-known people the notes provide some background information about their life and achievements.

Here are some general suggestions for discussion:

■ Do members of the group recognise the face? If so what do they know about the person?

■ Did they like or dislike the person—and why?

■ Other famous people in related fields, i.e. if the photograph shows a famous cricketer—other famous cricketers they admired.

■ Famous events or achievements associated with the person, e.g. famous films or plays starred in.

Group members should be encouraged to make and discuss their own list of famous personalities.

Individuals may also have their own collection of material relating to specific topics, i.e. scrap books of sports personalities. Encourage people to bring these in to show the group to enable everyone to share their memories.

Louis Armstrong

Louis Armstrong was born in July 1900 into a very poor family. His grandparents had been slaves. After his birth his parents separated and he was brought up by his grandmother. After a haphazard schooling, he joined a street quartet. In 1913 he was arrested for firing a pistol into the air during the traditional New Orleans New Year celebrations and he was sent to a remand home. There he joined the school band and soon became the band leader. At 16 he earned his keep as a coalman and played the cornet in the bars around Stonyville at night. Then he met King Oliver, the man who taught him jazz and with whom he made his first recording. In 1925 he made the first of the Hot 5 recordings, one of the best jazz pieces of that era. During the next few years he played with many of the top bands and made countless records.

In the 1930s he moved from jazz to blues and became a stage and film personality. In 1947 he formed the first of the Armstrong All Star Groups and travelled all over the world. He made many film appearances, the most famous of which was "Hello Dolly", in which he sang for only one minute the title song "Hello Dolly". Armstrong was one of the greatest jazz musicians of all time. He continued to play until he suffered a heart attack in March 1971 and died 2 days after his 72nd birthday.

Arthur Askey

Arthur Askey was a small, much-loved music-hall comedian who entertained audiences with 'silly little songs'. He was born in Liverpool in 1900 and on leaving school became a Corporation clerk. He started his professional career at the age of 24 when he joined a touring concert party, with whom he stayed for the next 14 years.

By 1938 Askey was an enormous success on radio in Britain's first comedy series "Band Wagon". He used many catch phrases, such as "I thank you" and "Hello Playmates", and could raise laughter from references to "combs" and by his tongue-twisting songs about "busy, busy bees" and "impudent pixies". He made several films including "Bees in Paradise" and "Make Mine a Million". He also worked as an after-dinner entertainer in London, and appeared in musical comedies, at Palladium revues and at several Royal Command Performances.

In his 70s Askey could still project the image of the mischievous schoolboy which brought him fame in his earlier years.

Clement Attlee

Clement Attlee became the first Prime Minister of the British Labour Party with an independent majority. He was born in 1883 and educated at Oxford. Early in life he became devoted to the interests of the working class and worked in the East End of London from 1910 to 1913. His army service in Mesopotamia brought him the rank of Major. After the war he became Mayor of Stepney and entered Parliament in 1922. He held office in MacDonald's government but went into opposition with several of his colleagues when, because of the financial crisis of 1931, MacDonald formed a coalition.

Attlee was a loyal and efficient deputy to Churchill in the wartime coalition and after the 1945 election, he became Prime Minister with a large majority. Various nationalization projects and a series of measures which provided the basis of the welfare state are associated with Attlee's period of office.

Attlee received an earldom and retired from the House of Commons in 1955. He spoke often in the House of Lords. He died in 1967.

Roger Bannister

The most famous of all the athletic barriers, the 4-minute mile, went to Roger Bannister at Oxford on 6th May 1954. After long and careful preparations, his finishing time clipped 2 seconds from the previous world record. 1954, his final season, made up for his Olympic disappointment at Helsinki where he was a finalist 2 years earlier. Bannister's second epic race of 1954 was at the Empire Games in Vancouver on 7th August where he won a long-awaited duel with Landy, the second of the 4-minute milers. Both men finished in under 4 minutes. He then won the 1500-metre title at Berne on 29th August, the last race of his career.

Bannister raced sparingly during his career and stopped to concentrate on completing his medical studies. He went on to become a consultant physician neurologist. Following his chairmanship of the Sports Council, he was knighted in 1975.

Thomas Beecham

Born in 1879, Thomas Beecham became one of the country's most celebrated conductors. His father was a baronet and Beecham succeeded to the title in 1916. He studied at Oxford, but not formally in the Music School. He first appeared as a conductor in 1906; symphonic concerts given around this time included new works by Strauss and Delius.

As an operatic impresario, Beecham produced more than sixty works that were new to Britain, and in 1911 he took London by storm when he introduced Russian ballet. Other notable achievements during his life included founding the London Philharmonic Orchestra in 1932 and becoming Artistic Director of Covent Garden Opera in 1933.

It was said of Beecham that he could inspire any orchestra to heights that even the musicians themselves had not imagined they could reach. He was notable not only for the clarity of his interpretations, but also for his service to British music and musicians.

Clara Bow

Clara Bow was brought up in Brooklyn by a mentally disturbed mother. She had an unhappy childhood and escaped from it when she won a beauty competition, which began her career in films. She acted in "Beyond the Rainbow" in 1922 and within a year she was a star with Paramount. At the peak of her career in 1925 she was known as "The Hottest Jazz Baby in Films".

Clara became known as Hollywood's "It Girl" for her portrayal of a carefree, wide-eyed shop girl in the film "It" in 1927. In the 1920s it was thought that a girl with energy and vitality could always get on if she had "it". Clara capitalised on her reputation as a sex symbol in "Mantrap" and "Call Her Savage" in 1932.

Offstage she lived a life style that matched her screen image. Scandal in her private life hastened the end of her career after she made "Hoopla" in 1933. In retirement she put on weight alarmingly and became a recluse. She suffered from chronic insomnia and moved from sanatorium to sanatorium. She died of a heart attack in 1965.

Maria Callas

Greek by parentage and naturalization, Maria Callas was born in New York on 3rd December 1923. At 13 years old, her mother took her to Greece where she studied at the Athens Conservatory. She made her debut at Verona, Italy, in "La Gioconda" in 1947 and was soon famous throughout Italy. With her impressive voice and magnificent interpretative powers she was soon in demand, especially when rare and vocally taxing operas of the older school were revived.

Maria Callas became one of the greatest sopranos of the 20th century, singing in major opera houses throughout the world. Her marriage to her manager, Meneghini, ended after 10 years in 1959 and she became the centre of much publicity because of her association with Aristotle Onassis. Criticized for being fiery tempered and difficult to work with, the truth was that an exacting self-critical temperament and recurrent vocal troubles caused her increasing problems. She retired from the stage in 1965 but gave a highly successful series of master classes in New York in 1971 and also made extensive recital tours.

Neville Chamberlain

Neville Chamberlain was born in Edgbaston and educated at Rugby. He spent 7 years in the Bahamas as manager of his father's sisal plantation before he went into industry and local politics in Birmingham, where he became Lord Mayor in 1915. In 1918 he was elected Conservative MP for Birmingham.

Chamberlain succeeded Baldwin as Prime Minister in May 1937 and immediately faced a series of crises in foreign affairs, an area unfamiliar to him. He twice sought a settlement with Hitler and believed that by the Munich Agreement he had ensured "peace in our time". When Hitler occupied Czechoslovakian territories in 1939 he abandoned the Agreement and offered military alliances to Poland, Romania and Greece, then threatened by Mussolini. It was to honour Chamberlain's pledge to Poland that Britain went to war against Germany in 1939.

Mounting criticism from MPs of all parties forced Chamberlain to resign on 10th May 1940. Chamberlain was a most able and loyal politician and, although he was ill, he remained in the cabinet until 5 weeks before he died in November 1940.

Charlie Chaplin

Charlie Chaplin, born in 1889, was reared in poverty, and, like his parents, became a music hall performer. He joined the Keystone Studio and made his first film, "Make a Living", in 1914. This began his career as cinema's most celebrated comedian-actor. He was also well known in his role as director, producer, writer and interpreter of films. His most famous role was the Little Tramp, which highlighted social inequality, and he intermingled the pathos of the figure with humour. His parts usually required skilful acrobatics and he did all the stunts himself. Two of his best films were "The Gold Rush", 1925, and "The Great Dictator", 1940, which was his first all-talking film.

His personal life was somewhat troubled. He married 4 times and defended a paternity suit in 1944. He refused to accept US citizenship as he had been accused of Communist sympathies. He lived happily for many years in Switzerland with his wife and nine children. In 1972 he returned to the United States in triumph when he received a special award from the Academy of Motion Pictures, Arts & Sciences. He was knighted in 1975 at the age of 86 by Queen Elizabeth, and died in 1977.

Winston Churchill

Churchill held most of the high offices of state in Great Britain, was a member of Parliament for more than 60 years and served twice as Prime Minister. Born in 1874, he became a journalist and war correspondent and was elected to Parliament as a Conservative in 1900 but became a Liberal in 1904. He served under Lloyd George as Minister for Munitions in 1917. He lost his seat when the coalition fell in 1922. In 1939 the war broke out and Churchill was offered his old job as First Lord of the Admiralty.

In 1940 Chamberlain resigned and Churchill became Prime Minister. His main aim was to communicate to the British people, allies and oppressed people of occupied Europe his unshakable faith in ultimate victory. He lost power in 1945 when the Labour Party took office but by the end of 1951 he had his final term as Prime Minister. This time he was preoccupied with ensuring the Cold War between Russia and the West should not escalate into a nuclear holocaust. In 1953 he was knighted and that same year suffered a stroke. He died in 1965.

Maureen Connolly

Maureen Connolly was spotted playing tennis in San Diego by Wilbur Folson at the age of 11. He radically changed the style of her game when he persuaded her to change from left to right-handed. She also made remarkable progress under the guidance of top tennis coach, Eleanor 'Teach' Tennant. At 13 she was the youngest girl to win the American National Junior championships. In 1951, at only 16, she became America's youngest Wightman Cup player and 9 days later won the American championships.

Maureen won Wimbledon when she was only 17 and was given the nickname "Little Mo". She beat Doris Hart in a game that goes down as a Wimbledon classic in 1953. Little Mo went on to win the US title and became the first woman to win the Grand Slam in the same year. Having won Wimbledon and US titles three years running, as well as French and Australian titles, she was forced to retire at the age of only 21 after she broke her leg in a riding accident. She had a happy marriage with fellow American Norman Brinker. Maureen Connolly died in June 1969.

Noel Coward

Noel Coward was born on 16th December 1899 in Teddington, Middlesex, and grew up in suburban London. He started acting at the age of ten and at twenty was already appearing in one of his own productions. His first real success came at the age of 24 with "The Vortex", of which he was author, director and leading actor. He became the 'darling' of the 1920s; 1928 to 1934 were golden years with successes such as "Private Lives", "Bitter Sweet" and "Cavalcade". In 1941 he wrote "Blithe Spirit". During the second world war, he gave troop concerts as a cabaret entertainer.

In the 1950s his private and professional life suffered a depression, but in the 1960s the National Theatre production of "Hay Fever" brought about a Noel Coward Renaissance in his own lifetime. Noel Coward was knighted in 1970 and although he spent most of his later life abroad, he remained strongly attached to England.

Bing Crosby

Bing Crosby was born in 1904 in Washington and became the most popular singer in the United States between 1930 and 1950. In 1931 a radio show brought him national fame and a 3-year contract for five films with Paramount. In the 1930s he was in a series of films ranging from light musicals to a dramatic role in "Sing You Sinners" in 1938. In the following year he started making the popular "Road" films with Bob Hope.

Famous for his unique 'crooning' style, he made many records, including the world-wide best-seller "White Christmas". In films, his easy-going personality made him a box-office star. He made a total of 58 films and won an Academy Award for "Going My Way" in 1944. His film career ended with a disastrous remake of "Stagecoach" in 1966.

Crosby remarried in 1957 and a second chance at family life proved happier than the first. He died in 1977 on the golf course. He had won a game and turning to acknowledge the applause, he suffered a fatal heart attack.

Charles de Gaulle

As a child, Charles de Gaulle dreamed of becoming a soldier and saving France. In the First World War he showed himself an officer of extraordinary courage. During the Second World War he mounted the only 2 offensives to be carried out by the French army during the battle of France, though these failed for lack of resources. He rallied the Free French, persuading them to continue fighting after defeat by Germany, using England as the base for continued French resistance. Following liberation he was recognised Head of the Provisional French Government. In 1946 he resigned rather than meet opposition demands to reduce military expenditure. In 1958 he was recalled to deal with Algerian independence problems and was elected President.

In 1960 he gave France an independent nuclear military force and tried to restore her status as a great power. During the 1960s he succeeded in stabilising the economy, industry and social life of France but at the expense of democratic liberties. In 1966 he was re-elected President for another 7-year term, but after a year of industrial unrest and student riots, he appealed to the country for a fresh mandate but was defeated in a constitutional referendum and retired in 1969. De Gaulle died unexpectedly from a heart attack in 1970.

Marlene Dietrich

Marlene Dietrich was a screen goddess worshipped by everyone from her director downwards. The daughter of a Prussian police officer, she studied music and then acted in the theatre. She had made over a dozen films when she was discovered by Sternberg, who starred her as the femme fatale Lola-Lola in "The Blue Angel". After this she was offered a contract in Hollywood, where she made six more films with Sternberg before they went their separate ways. Her subsequent films were less enticing, but the spoof western "Destry Rides Again" kept her a star.

Marlene Dietrich tirelessly entertained the allied troops during the second world war. She also gave some excellent performances in "Stage Fright", "Rancho Notorious", "Witness for the Prosecution" and "Touch of Evil". She was still beautiful and glamorous when she embarked on a series of famous live concert tours at the age of almost sixty. After her disappointment with "Just a Gigolo", she finally retired from films at the age of 78.

Richard Dimbleby

Richard Dimbleby was a broadcaster, author, newspaper director, editor and film producer. Born in 1913 into a newspaper family, his grounding in journalism came with the family firm. At the age of 21 he became news editor of the London "Advertisers' Weekly". In 1936 the BBC appointed him its first full-time observer in what was then a small experimental news department. He visited many countries and broadcasted on major news events including state visits to France and Canada.

With his 'star quality' he could do little wrong and his profession, show business and newspapers all crowded awards upon him. He changed to the media of television with a series called "London Town". Within 3 years he was once again first in the field. In 1953 he was the commentator at the coronation of Elizabeth II. He died in 1965.

Gracie Fields

Gracie Fields was born Grace Stansfield in 1898. She worked in a cotton mill and as a draper's assistant, but, encouraged by her mother, appeared in amateur shows from the age of eight. Turning professional, she joined a touring revue, where she met and married her first husband. In 1923 the review "Mr Tower of London" came to the West End and she became an overnight star.

The film "Sally" heralded the most successful decade of her career and she was awarded the CBE. At the outbreak of the Second World War she gave very popular concerts to the troops in France. When she married her second husband and left for America in 1940 public opinion swung against her though she raised over £1,500,000 for the war effort. In 1950, after the death of her second husband, she retired to Capri where in 1952 she married for the third time.

Gracie returned to England for occasional concerts and was warmly greeted at the Royal Command Performances, where she made a total of ten appearances. She wrote an autobiography "Sing as We Go" and in 1979 was created a DBE.

W C Fields

W.C. Fields was an eccentric genius who created brilliant comedy. It was difficult to separate the characters he played—cheats, drunks, con-men—from the real Fields. His art was derived from his experience: he ran away from home at the age of 12 and lived rough. Dogs, bankers, women and children were the main butt of his humour.

Born in Philadelphia in 1879, W.C. Fields first went into show business as a juggler. By the time he was 25 he was an international star. His first film was "Pool Sharks" in 1915. In the 1920s he signed with Paramount but was dropped because of his difficult character. It was not until 1932 that he regained his position in Hollywood and appeared in several films, notably "International House" in 1933 and "David Copperfield" in 1935.

Fields' last film was "Never Give a Sucker an Even Break" made in 1941. He died on Christmas Day, 1946.

Margot Fonteyn

Margot Fonteyn's career as a prima ballerina spans several decades. She was born in Surrey in 1919 and as a child travelled with her parents to North America and China. She attended the Sadler's Wells Ballet School. Her first performance was as a snowflake in Tchaikovsky's "Nutcracker" at Sadler's Wells in 1934. Due to the high standard of her performance she was picked out to succeed Alicia Markova as the company's principal ballerina and within five years she had danced "Giselle", "Swan Lake" and "The Sleeping Beauty". She was chosen to interpret the ballets of Frederick Ashton, who joined the Royal Ballet in 1935.

Margot Fonteyn's partnership with Rudolf Nureyev gave her a new lease on her career at an age when most dancers are thinking of retiring. She became a 'jet set' ballerina, appearing with many partners and companies all over the world.

Greta Garbo

Greta Garbo, born in Stockholm, Sweden, is often called the greatest romantic star in film history. She appeared originally in publicity films but felt she was wasting her time posing for cheap pictures. Although she needed the money, she realized it was not much compared with the earnings of other actresses and in 1927 she went on strike. Finally, her employers, the huge Hollywood corporation MGM, gave way to her, knowing what potential she had. This alone gave her tremendous prestige in her later acting life.

She appeared in many silent films with torrid love scenes and melodramatic plots that were aimed at popular audiences. When sound came into films, she began to get more worthy and interesting roles. The first film she acted in, "Anna Christie", in 1930, caused great excitement. Her voice was deep, rich and heavily accented and matched the aura of mystery that surrounded her. She went on to make many successful films, including "Grand Hotel" in 1931 and "Anna Karenina" in 1935.

David Lloyd George

Lloyd George was Prime Minister from 1916 to 1922 and during his life as a politician led many social reforms. He was a forceful leader during the First World War. Welsh in background, Lloyd George was born in Manchester in 1863. He was elected to Parliament as a Liberal in 1890, the beginning of a 55-year career at Westminster. He acquired recognition by standing up for the interests of Welsh non-conformists and was considered to be very unorthodox. In 1911 he pioneered the National Health Insurance Act, which together with the Old Age Pension Act, laid the foundation for the British welfare state.

Lloyd George became Prime Minister in 1916. Often held to be the man who won the war, he exploited this reputation to win a huge election victory. When the Liberal/Conservative coalition fell in 1922, he never again held office. He was awarded an earldom shortly before his death in 1945.

John Gielgud

An actor with a beautiful voice which he uses with subtlety and grace, John Gielgud achieved great distinction playing Shakespearean roles. He has appeared in and directed countless productions on radio, television, in films and on stage in plays such as "Romeo and Juliet", "Hamlet", "The Merchant of Venice", "The Importance of Being Earnest", and as director and actor in "Richard of Bordeaux". In 1933 he directed and starred in an even more triumphant "Hamlet".

He appeared in many films, but most post-war parts were unworthy of the actor with exceptions such as "The Good Companions", "The Secret Agent" and most recently "Providence". He also narrated for many films. many films.

In the 1960s he toured widely with a solo Shakespearean recital "The Ages of Man" and in 1975 appeared in Harold Pinter's "No Man's Land" with Sir Ralph Richardson. One of the greatest English stage actors of his time, John Gielgud was knighted in 1953.

Will Hay

Will Hay was one of the most successful British music-hall stars to enter films. Before he was 20 he gave up an engineering apprenticeship to try his luck in the music halls and after the First World War he established himself with the comedy sketch "The Fourth Form at St. Michael's". He developed this act during 10 years in films and portrayed a disreputable, seedy character with a pair of pince-nez and a shifty look. His films were not particularly well made, leaning heavily on poor verbal humour, but were often saved by the contrasting characters of the three leads: Hay was the figure of tatty authority, Moffatt played the insolent Cockney fat boy and Moore Marriott was the shrill and toothless old man. Their masterpiece is "Oh! Mr. Porter!" about a crumbling branch-line station.

Off screen Will Hay was a solitary man who rarely gave interviews. He preferred to live apart from show business. He died in 1949.

Bob Hope

Bob Hope was born in London in 1903. When he was 4 his family emigrated to Ohio and later he became an American radio, film and television comedian. After appearing in Vaudeville and on Broadway as a song-and-dance man, he achieved fame in the 1930s in films. "Road to Singapore" in 1940 launched him on his long partnership with Bing Crosby. The humour was uncomplicated and reassuring, exactly what a wartime audience needed. The film allowed Hope to demonstrate his non-stop wise-cracking. Many writers helped create his distinctive comic personality: a brash, egocentric wit who specialized in topical jokes.

During the war Bob Hope undertook heavy tours of Europe and the Far East in order to entertain the troops.

25

Len Hutton

Most people will remember Len Hutton for his record score of 364 runs in the England v Australia test match in 1938 and as the second man ever to be knighted for his services to cricket. He is also one of a handful of cricketers to have made a century on his test debut against Australia and one of a select band, too, who have made over 100 centuries in first-class cricket. In June 1949 he broke the record for the number of runs made in a month—1,294—a record that still stands today.

He was a first-class batsman, even though his left arm was shorter and weaker than his right. For years he was Australia's tormentor, but played in a very weak batting side which resulted in many defeats for the English team. This was highlighted in the 1950 to 51 series which England lost, although Hutton's average was better than the best of his Australian adversaries.

Len Hutton captained the English team 23 times. In retirement he became a successful businessman and for a time he also selected cricketers to play for England.

26

Amy Johnson

Born in Hull in 1904, Amy Johnson took a degree in Economics, then began flying in 1928. Two years later, she made the solo flight half way round the world, which caused the press to hail her as 'Queen of the Air'. With no financial backing, she gained the Ground Engineers Licence and studied courses in meteorology, direction finding and signalling. Her aim was to fly solo to Australia. She set off from Croydon on 5th May 1930 in her biplane "Jason", but encountered weather problems, thereby suffering damage to the propellor and undercarriage, and was forced to land near Rangoon. Her aircraft repaired, she finally flew into Darwin, Australia, on 24th May 1930 to a rapturous welcome.

Despite a supreme command of the air, she crashed and was killed at the age of 37 whilst flying an aeroplane to Kidlington.

Joe Louis

Born Joseph Barrow, May 1914, Joe Louis became the light heavyweight Golden Gloves boxing champion at the age of only 20, and turned professional the same year. His deceptive style was soon recognised throughout the United States as he won his first 27 fights. But his next fight against former World Champion Max Schmeling in June 1936 ended with Louis being knocked out in the 12th round. Louis had to wait 2 years to get his chance to make amends for that defeat and did so by stopping Schmeling in only 2 minutes 4 seconds in round 1.

A year to the day before his return with Schmeling, Louis had won the World Heavyweight title in the 8th round against holder James J. Braddock. He defended the title 25 times until his retirement in 1949, with only 3 men going the distance with him. After retirement, Louis fought exhibition fights only, until he was persuaded to fight Ezzard Charles for the World Boxing Association world title, but at 36 years of age, he was outpointed by Charles. His career finally ended when Rocky Marciano knocked him out in October 1951 and he retired.

Vera Lynn

Vera Lynn was born in East Ham, London, in 1917 and began singing in public at the age of 7. She joined a dancing troupe at 11 and from the age of 15 was involved in running a small dancing school. In 1935 she began recording with Joe Loss and joined the Charlie Lunz band. She was so popular that she went solo.

During the second world war she was known as the "Forces Sweetheart" with her golden hair, slim body and charming smile. She sang simple lyrics in an unsophisticated manner and united and inspired the nation in a series of now legendary broadcasts. She chose to go to Burma, one of the toughest areas, to entertain the troops and carry on the morale boosting she had begun through broadcasting.
well as in cabaret and variety shows all over the world. She appeared in seven Royal Command performances and received many honours, including the DBE in 1975 and Freedom of the City of London in 1978.

Harold Macmillan

Harold Macmillan held a succession of ministerial posts during the early 1950s and became Prime Minister in 1957. He was educated at Eton and Oxford and became a Conservative member in 1924. He held various positions in government and was active in trying to improve relations with the USA strained by the Suez crisis. He also tried to strengthen Britain's ties with Europe by joining the EEC, but was rebuffed by de Gaulle who vetoed British entry in 1963.

In 1959 Macmillan led his party to a landslide victory because of the healthy state of the British economy. In 1963 he resigned because of bad health. He retired from the government in 1964. He has written six volumes of his memoirs to date.

Groucho Marx

Groucho Marx, born in 1890 in New York City, is remembered primarily for his comic role as the bushy-browed, leering, cigar-smoking leader of the trio "The Marx Brothers". He starred with his two brothers, Harpo and Chico, and they became famous for the way they attacked middle-class morality. They specialized in slapstick comedy that resulted in spontaneous lunacy whenever possible.

In 1924 the Marx Brothers moved on to Broadway musical revues with "I'll Say She Is", followed by "Animal Crackers" in 1928 and the classic "Duck Soup" in 1933.

The team split up in 1941. Groucho did well from then on as a solo performer, mainly as the aggressive host of radio and television quiz shows; he hosted "You Bet Your Life", a popular show that ran from 1947 until 1961. Groucho married for the third time at the age of 64. He died in 1977.

Stanley Matthews

Stanley Matthews was born in Hanley, Stoke-on-Trent in 1915, the son of a well known boxer. He started playing football with home-town side Stoke City, as a brilliant schoolboy prodigy, and became known as 'The Wizard of the Dribble'. In 1947 he transferred to Blackpool Football Club for £11,500. After losing two F.A. cup finals, he achieved a life-time ambition when Blackpool beat Bolton in the 1952-53 F.A. cup final, which became known as the "Matthews' Final". He then returned to Stoke City, helping them back into the First Division, and was still playing First Division football at the age of 50.

Stanley Matthews first played football for England in 1935 and 22 years later in 1957 had played a total of 54 international games. Although not a prolific goal scorer himself, he was the greatest goal provider in the history of football. He will always be remembered for his ball control and body swerve. One of football's greatest legends, Matthews received a knighthood whilst still playing.

Marilyn Monroe

Born Norma Jean Baker in Los Angeles on 1 June 1926, Marilyn Monroe's childhood dream was to become a movie star. In spite of a troubled childhood and several marriages, she did become a very famous and glamorous actress.

Her route to success began in 1944 when she drifted into photographic modelling. This led to a contract with 20th Century Fox and this is when she changed her name. Her first decent parts were in "The Asphalt Jungle" and "All About Eve", and she secured her stardom in 1953 with "Gentlemen Prefer Blondes". Her most memorable performance was probably in "Some Like It Hot", one of Hollywood's most successful comedies. Arthur Miller, her third husband, wrote the screenplay for her final completed film "The Misfits", in which she starred with Clark Gable in 1961. She died in 1962 at the age of 36.

Bernard Montgomery

Known as Monty, Bernard Montgomery was born in London in 1887 and spent much of his childhood in Tasmania where his father was a Bishop. Educated at St Paul's and Sandhurst, he became Britain's most successful 20th century General. He made his reputation with the Eighth Army in North Africa, Sicily and Italy. He commanded Allied troops during the Normandy landings in 1944 and played the decisive part in turning back the German counter-attack in the Ardennes. In May 1945 he formally accepted the surrender of all German forces in North West Europe at Lüneburg Heath.

A non-smoker and teetotaller, Monty set his men an outstanding example of physical fitness and mental alertness. From 1946 to 1948 he was Chief of Imperial General Staff, and Deputy Supreme Commander of NATO forces in Europe from 1951 to 1958, when he finally retired from the army. He died at home in Hampshire on 24th March 1976.

Emmeline Pankhurst

Emmeline Pankhurst is remembered primarily for her role as a militant suffragette, in particular for her attempt to gain the vote for women. She was born into a family of English abolitionists in 1867 and became a social activist, determined to end the exploitation and misery she saw around her. This led to the realisation that men and women must have the power to determine their own existence, and that the vote for both sexes was necessary to achieve this. In 1903 she founded the 'Women's Social and Political Union', which became the largest militant women's group in England. Their motto was "Deeds, not Words".

In the years that followed, she was involved with many political promises and betrayals, and took part in peaceful demonstrations that turned into riots. There were beatings, over 1000 women were imprisoned, and there were many cases of forced feeding. To achieve their aims, the Union took to deliberate violence, arson and even bombings. Eventually, in 1918, women over the age of 30 were given the vote, but it was not until 1928, the year of Emmeline Pankhurst's death, that women achieved full equality with respect to the vote.

Sylvia Peters

Sylvia Peters was the most famous face on British television from 1946 to 1955. She was the BBC announcer of post-war years and the first woman television celebrity.

Like radio, television started very shakily. In 1929 the BBC staged an experimental television broadcast. The men who appeared were so heavily made-up that they looked like clowns; they spoke into the microphone first and then turned silently to face the camera. Baird was overtaken by Marconi and EMI who devised a greatly superior television system.

Television made little progress until after the Second World War. The highlight came with the Coronation of Queen Elizabeth II in 1953. The BBC televised the great pageant in all its splendour. About 20 million people watched the ceremony on television. Viewing parties were held in private houses and thousands of people bought tickets to watch television screens set up in hotels, cinemas and shops.

Ronald Reagan

Born in 1911, Ronald Wilson Reagan was a well-known actor before he entered politics. After graduating from college in 1932 he worked as a radio sportscaster until 1937, when he signed up with Warner Brothers film studio. He worked with them for 13 years. His first major film role was playing opposite Bette Davis in "Dark Victory". During his career in Hollywood he acted in more than 50 films and served six terms as president of the Screen Actors' Guild. He married for the first time in 1940. Reagan focused his career increasingly on television and starred in several weekly programmes, such as "The General Electric Theater".

In middle age, he played a few tough western roles before he entered the world of politics. He married his second wife, Nancy Davis, in 1952. In his new political life, Reagan moved from liberal to conservative in his views and from Democrat to Republican in party. He was elected Governor of California in 1966, the start of his future life in politics, and he became President of the United States in 1980.

Edward G. Robinson

Born in Romania in 1893, Edward G. Robinson became one of the major Hollywood figures in the 1930s. He was short and dynamic, with a distinctive voice, and specialized in gangster parts, although he later proved to be equally good at comedy and character roles. His first really successful film was "Little Caesar" in 1930.

In 1927 he married and set up home with his wife in Beverley Hills. He built up a superb art collection which he valued above everything. He made over 50 films in the next 20 years. His son, born in 1933, was unstable and awkward and Robinson was forever paying fines and getting him out of trouble after drinking episodes.

In the early 1950s Robinson was unjustly labelled a Communist sympathizer and was blacklisted from the studios. Eventually he was cleared of this charge and made several more or less successful films. After divorcing his first wife, he married a girl 26 years his junior. This started a much happier phase in his life. In 1973 he was shown on his deathbed holding an Oscar, in recognition of his achievement in films.

Joan Sutherland

Joan Sutherland was born in 1926 in Sydney, Australia. She made her debut as a soprano at Covent Garden in "The Magic Flute" in 1952, having sung in "Dido and Aeneas" in 1947 in Australia and in many oratorio broadcasts. She remained resident soprano for 7 years. The first person to realize her potential as a dramatic singer was her husband, conductor Richard Bonynge. After her performance of "Lucia di Lammermoor" in 1959, she sang in every major opera house in the world.

She has performed regularly in the USA, Europe and Australia. Her roles have included Bellini's "Norma", "Elvira" and "Beatrice di Tenda", "Violetta" and a most successful entry into comedy, "The Daughter of the Regiment". She has a unique voice and has made many records. She was awarded the CBE in 1961, the AC in 1975 and the DBE in 1979.

Shirley Temple

Shirley Temple was the great child sensation of the 1930s. Born in California in 1928, her mother was determined she should become an actress. Before she was four years old, she had moved from dancing classes into films. She was an adorable, golden-haired child with the timing and reactions of an adult. She appeared completely natural on screen. Her first film was "The Red-Haired Alibi" in 1932; in 1934 she won a contract with Fox and starred in "Little Miss Marker". She was America's top star between 1935 and 1938.

She married at 17, divorced at 21 and re-married a year later. She retired from acting in 1949 after a series of unremarkable teenage films. Her career as a diplomat started in the late 1960s when she ran as a Republican candidate for Congress. She became a Nixon appointee as representative to the United Nations in 1968. She also acted as American Ambassador to Ghana and Chief of Protocol in the Ford Administration from 1976 to 1977.

Rudolph Valentino

The son of a veterinary doctor, Rudolph Valentino was born in 1895 in Italy. After taking an Agriculturalist's Diploma he set off for America in 1913 to seek work as a gardener. He learned to dance in the dance halls and cafés of New York, while working as an apprentice landscape gardener in Central Park. The Head Waiter at Maxims hired him as a dancer and so began his professional career.

After touring with a musical comedy troupe, he went to Los Angeles and worked occasionally in Hollywood as an extra. His first triumph came when he was selected for the role of Julio in "The Four Horsemen of the Apocalypse". He leapt from obscurity to fame almost overnight. Early pictures include "Camilla", "Blood and Sand" and "Beyond the Rocks", in which he appeared opposite Gloria Swanson. He gained his nickname from the film "The Sheik" at the age of 26. His last film "The Son of the Sheik" opened in New York in July 1926.